HYPOTHYROIDISM DIET COOKBOOK FOR BEGINNERS

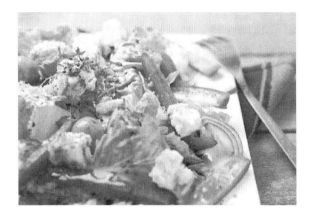

DR. JESSICA SMITH

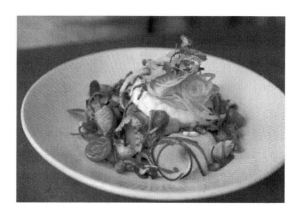

TABLE OF CONTENTS

CHAPTER ONE

How to Use this Cookbook

Familiarize Yourself with the Basics: Start by reading the introductory sections of the cookbook. Understand what hypothyroidism is, how it affects your body, and the role of diet in managing the condition.

Review the Food Guidelines: Pay close attention to the dietary guidelines provided in the cookbook. Look for recommendations on foods to include and foods to avoid for optimal thyroid health.

Browse Through Recipes: Take some time to browse through the recipe sections of the cookbook. Get a sense of the variety of dishes available, including breakfasts, lunches, dinners, snacks, and desserts.

Make a Shopping List: Select a few recipes that appeal to you and make a list of ingredients needed. Check your pantry to see what you already have and jot down the items you need to buy.

Meal Planning: Plan your meals for the week using the recipes from the cookbook. Consider factors like convenience, variety, and nutritional balance when selecting recipes for each day.

Preparation: Before you start cooking, read through the recipe instructions carefully. Gather all the necessary ingredients and equipment to ensure a smooth cooking process.

Cooking: Follow the step-by-step instructions provided in the cookbook to prepare your chosen recipes. Take your time and enjoy the cooking process.

Portion Control: Pay attention to portion sizes to ensure you're not overeating. Use measuring cups and spoons if needed, especially when dealing with ingredients like grains and fats.

Storage and Leftovers: If you have leftovers, store them properly in airtight containers in the refrigerator or freezer. This allows you to have convenient, healthy meals on hand for busy days.

Enjoy Your Meals: Sit down, savor your delicious creations, and pay attention to how your body feels after eating. Notice any changes in energy levels, digestion, or overall well-being as you incorporate thyroid-friendly recipes into your diet.

By following these simple steps, you can effectively utilize a hypothyroidism diet cookbook to plan and prepare nutritious meals that support thyroid health and overall wellness.

Understanding Hypothyroidism Diet for Beginners

Understanding the hypothyroidism diet is essential for individuals managing this condition, as diet plays a significant role in supporting thyroid function and overall health.

Hypothyroidism occurs when the thyroid gland doesn't produce enough thyroid hormone, leading to symptoms such as fatigue, weight gain, and sensitivity to cold.

While medication is often necessary for treatment, adopting a hypothyroidism diet can complement medical management and alleviate symptoms.

The primary goal of a hypothyroidism diet is to provide adequate nutrients that support thyroid function and minimize foods that may interfere with hormone production or absorption. Key components of a hypothyroidism diet include:

Iodine-Rich Foods: Iodine is essential for thyroid hormone production. Including iodine-rich foods like seafood, seaweed, and iodized salt can help support thyroid health.

Selenium: Selenium is another important nutrient for thyroid function and can be found in foods like Brazil nuts, eggs, and sunflower seeds.

Balanced Macronutrients: A well-rounded diet with adequate protein, healthy fats, and complex carbohydrates supports overall health and metabolism.

Limiting Goitrogens: Some foods, known as goitrogens, can interfere with thyroid function when consumed in large amounts. These include cruciferous vegetables like broccoli, cabbage, and kale. While these foods are nutritious, they should be eaten in moderation and cooked to reduce their goitrogenic properties.

Avoiding Excess Sugar and Processed Foods: High-sugar and processed foods can disrupt blood sugar levels and contribute to inflammation, which may negatively impact thyroid function.

Understanding and implementing these dietary principles can help individuals with hypothyroidism better manage their condition and improve their overall quality of life.

However, it's essential to work with a healthcare professional or registered dietitian to tailor dietary recommendations to individual needs and ensure optimal thyroid health.

Principles of Hypothyroidism Diet for Beginners

The principles of a hypothyroidism diet revolve around supporting thyroid function, managing symptoms, and promoting overall health and well-being.

While there isn't a one-size-fits-all approach, several key principles can guide dietary choices for individuals with hypothyroidism:

Balanced Macronutrients: A hypothyroidism diet should include a balance of macronutrients, including protein, carbohydrates, and fats.

Protein-rich foods like lean meats, poultry, fish, legumes, and tofu provide essential amino acids necessary for thyroid hormone production and metabolism.

Complex carbohydrates from whole grains, fruits, and vegetables provide sustained energy levels, while healthy fats from sources like avocados, nuts, seeds, and olive oil support hormone production and absorption.

Iodine and Selenium: Adequate intake of iodine and selenium is crucial for thyroid health. Iodine is a key component of thyroid hormones, while selenium is necessary for the conversion of inactive thyroid hormone (T4) to its active form (T3).

Including iodine-rich foods like seaweed, fish, dairy products, and iodized salt, as well as selenium-rich foods like Brazil nuts, eggs, and seafood, can support thyroid function.

Limiting Goitrogens: Some foods contain compounds known as goitrogens, which can interfere with thyroid function when consumed in large amounts. These include cruciferous vegetables like broccoli, cabbage, and kale.

While these foods offer numerous health benefits, cooking them can help reduce their goitrogenic properties.

Avoiding Excess Sugar and Processed Foods: High-sugar and processed foods can disrupt blood sugar levels and contribute to inflammation, which may negatively impact thyroid function.

Limiting intake of refined carbohydrates, sugary snacks, and processed foods can help stabilize blood sugar levels and support overall health.

Individualized Approach: It's essential to recognize that each person's nutritional needs and preferences may vary.

Consulting with a healthcare professional or registered dietitian can help individuals develop a personalized hypothyroidism diet plan that meets their specific needs and goals while supporting thyroid health and overall well-being.

Benefits of Hypothyroidism Diet for Beginners

Adopting a hypothyroidism diet can offer numerous benefits for individuals managing this condition.

By focusing on nutrient-rich foods and making dietary adjustments tailored to support thyroid health, individuals with hypothyroidism can experience improved symptoms and overall well-being. Some of the key benefits of a hypothyroidism diet include:

Supporting Thyroid Function: A hypothyroidism diet provides essential nutrients like iodine, selenium, and zinc necessary for optimal thyroid function.

By including foods rich in these nutrients, such as seafood, Brazil nuts, and whole grains, individuals can support thyroid hormone production and metabolism.

Managing Symptoms: Many symptoms of hypothyroidism, such as fatigue, weight gain, and constipation, can be alleviated or managed through dietary modifications.

For example, incorporating fiber-rich foods like fruits, vegetables, and whole grains can help promote regular bowel movements and alleviate constipation commonly associated with hypothyroidism.

Balancing Blood Sugar Levels: A hypothyroidism diet emphasizes whole, nutrient-dense foods and limits refined carbohydrates and sugary snacks. This approach can help stabilize blood sugar levels and prevent spikes and crashes in energy, supporting overall energy levels and mood stability.

Promoting Weight Management: Hypothyroidism can contribute to weight gain or difficulty losing weight due to a slowed metabolism.

A hypothyroidism diet focuses on nutrient-dense, low-calorie foods that support metabolism and energy production, making it easier to manage weight and achieve weight loss goals.

Reducing Inflammation: Certain dietary factors, such as processed foods and excessive sugar intake, can contribute to inflammation in the body, which may exacerbate symptoms of hypothyroidism.

A hypothyroidism diet emphasizes anti-inflammatory foods like fruits, vegetables, fatty fish, and nuts, which can help reduce inflammation and promote overall health.

Overall, adopting a hypothyroidism diet can offer a range of benefits, from supporting thyroid function and managing symptoms to promoting overall health and well-being.

By making mindful dietary choices and focusing on nutrient-rich foods, individuals with hypothyroidism can optimize their health and improve their quality of life.

Tips on Hypothyroidism Diet for Beginners

Managing hypothyroidism through diet involves making thoughtful choices to support thyroid health and overall well-being. Here are some essential tips for navigating a hypothyroidism diet:

Focus on Nutrient-Dense Foods: Emphasize whole, nutrient-dense foods such as fruits, vegetables, lean proteins, whole grains, and healthy fats. These foods provide essential vitamins, minerals, and antioxidants that support thyroid function and overall health.

Include Iodine-Rich Foods: Iodine is crucial for thyroid hormone production. Incorporate iodine-rich foods such as seafood (e.g., fish, seaweed), dairy products, and iodized salt into your diet to ensure adequate intake.

Prioritize Selenium: Selenium is essential for thyroid hormone metabolism. Include selenium-rich foods like Brazil nuts, sunflower seeds, eggs, and seafood in your diet to support thyroid function.

Limit Goitrogenic Foods: Some foods contain compounds known as goitrogens, which can interfere with thyroid function when consumed in large amounts. These include cruciferous vegetables like broccoli, cabbage, and kale. While these foods offer health benefits, cooking them can help reduce their goitrogenic properties.

Moderate Soy Intake: Soy contains compounds called isoflavones that may interfere with thyroid function, particularly when consumed in large amounts. Limit soy intake and opt for fermented soy products like tempeh and miso, which may have less of an impact on thyroid health.

Balance Carbohydrates: Aim for a balanced intake of carbohydrates from whole grains, fruits, and vegetables. Complex carbohydrates provide sustained energy levels and support metabolism, while minimizing refined carbohydrates and sugars can help stabilize blood sugar levels.

Stay Hydrated: Drink plenty of water throughout the day to support hydration and overall health. Proper hydration is essential for metabolism, digestion, and detoxification processes.

Work with a Healthcare Professional: Consult with a healthcare professional or registered dietitian who specializes in thyroid health. They can provide personalized guidance and support to help you optimize your diet for managing hypothyroidism effectively.

By incorporating these tips into your daily routine, you can create a balanced and nourishing hypothyroidism diet that supports thyroid health and promotes overall wellness.

Guidelines for Hypothyroidism Diet for Beginners

Navigating a hypothyroidism diet requires adherence to specific guidelines to support thyroid function and alleviate symptoms associated with the condition. Here are essential guidelines to follow:

Balanced Macronutrients: Ensure your diet includes a balance of macronutrients, including proteins, carbohydrates, and fats.

Opt for lean proteins such as poultry, fish, and legumes, complex carbohydrates from whole grains, fruits, and vegetables, and healthy fats from sources like avocados, nuts, seeds, and olive oil.

Iodine-Rich Foods: Incorporate iodine-rich foods like seafood, seaweed, dairy products, and iodized salt into your diet to support thyroid hormone production.

Selenium: Include selenium-rich foods such as Brazil nuts, eggs, sunflower seeds, and seafood to support thyroid function and hormone metabolism.

Limit Goitrogenic Foods: While nutritious, certain foods like cruciferous vegetables (e.g., broccoli, cabbage, kale) contain goitrogens that can interfere with thyroid function. Consume these foods in moderation and consider cooking them to reduce their goitrogenic properties.

Moderate Soy Intake: Soy contains compounds that may affect thyroid function, particularly when consumed in large amounts. Limit soy intake and choose fermented soy products like tempeh and miso instead.

Manage Sugar and Processed Foods: Minimize consumption of refined carbohydrates and sugary snacks, as they can disrupt blood sugar levels and contribute to inflammation, impacting thyroid function.

Stay Hydrated: Drink plenty of water to support hydration and facilitate metabolic processes in the body.

Consult with a Healthcare Professional: Work with a healthcare professional or registered dietitian who specializes in thyroid health to develop a personalized hypothyroidism diet plan tailored to your individual needs and preferences.

By adhering to these guidelines and making informed dietary choices, individuals with hypothyroidism can effectively manage their condition and improve overall well-being.

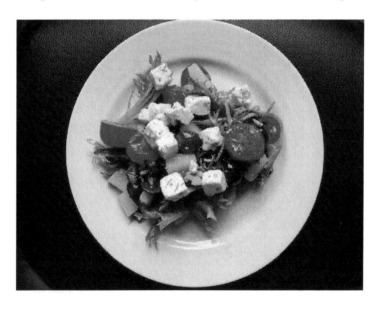

CHAPTER TWO

Hypothyroidism Diet Recipes for Beginners

1. Veggie Omelette

Ingredients:

- 2 eggs
- 1/4 cup diced bell peppers
- 1/4 cup diced tomatoes
- 1/4 cup chopped spinach
- Salt and pepper to taste
- 1 teaspoon olive oil

Instructions:

- Heat olive oil in a non-stick skillet over medium heat.
- In a bowl, whisk eggs until well beaten. Season with salt and pepper.
- Pour eggs into the skillet and swirl to spread evenly.
- Cook for 1-2 minutes until the edges start to set.
- Sprinkle bell peppers, tomatoes, and spinach evenly over one half of the omelette.
- Fold the other half of the omelette over the veggies.

> Cook for another 1-2 minutes until the veggies are heated through and the eggs are cooked.

> Slide the omelette onto a plate and serve hot.

Health Benefits:

> This omelette is packed with protein from eggs and loaded with nutrients from veggies like bell peppers, tomatoes, and spinach, providing essential vitamins and minerals to support thyroid health.

Preparation Time: 10 minutes

2. Greek Yogurt Parfait

Ingredients:

> 1/2 cup Greek yogurt
> 1/4 cup granola
> 1/4 cup mixed berries (such as strawberries, blueberries, raspberries)
> 1 tablespoon honey or maple syrup (optional)

Instructions:

> In a glass or bowl, layer Greek yogurt, granola, and mixed berries.
> Drizzle honey or maple syrup on top if desired.

- ➤ Repeat layers if making multiple servings.
- ➤ Serve immediately.

Health Benefits:

- ➤ Greek yogurt provides protein and probiotics, while granola offers fiber and healthy carbohydrates. Berries are rich in antioxidants, vitamins, and minerals, supporting overall health and thyroid function.

Preparation Time: 5 minutes

3. Quinoa Breakfast Bowl

Ingredients:

- ➤ 1/2 cup cooked quinoa
- ➤ 1/4 cup sliced avocado
- ➤ 1/4 cup diced tomatoes
- ➤ 1/4 cup steamed spinach
- ➤ 1 poached egg
- ➤ Salt and pepper to taste

Instructions:

- ➤ In a bowl, layer cooked quinoa, sliced avocado, diced tomatoes, and steamed spinach.

- ➤ Top with a poached egg.
- ➤ Season with salt and pepper to taste.
- ➤ Serve warm.

Health Benefits:

- ➤ Quinoa is a nutrient-dense whole grain that provides fiber, protein, and essential minerals like iron and magnesium. Avocado adds healthy fats, while tomatoes and spinach offer vitamins and antioxidants to support thyroid health.

Preparation Time: 15 minutes

4. Banana Nut Overnight Oats

Ingredients:

- ➤ 1/2 cup rolled oats
- ➤ 1/2 cup unsweetened almond milk
- ➤ 1/2 ripe banana, mashed
- ➤ 1 tablespoon chopped nuts (such as almonds, walnuts)
- ➤ 1 teaspoon honey or maple syrup (optional)
- ➤ Pinch of cinnamon (optional)

Instructions:

> In a jar or container, combine rolled oats, almond milk, mashed banana, chopped nuts, honey or maple syrup (if using), and cinnamon (if using).
> Stir well to combine.
> Cover and refrigerate overnight.
> In the morning, give the oats a stir and enjoy cold or warm.

Health Benefits:

> Rolled oats are a good source of fiber and complex carbohydrates, providing sustained energy and supporting digestive health.
> Banana adds natural sweetness and potassium, while nuts offer healthy fats and protein to keep you satisfied until lunch.

Preparation Time: 5 minutes (plus overnight soaking)

5. Spinach and Feta Breakfast Wrap

Ingredients:

> 1 whole wheat tortilla
> 2 eggs, scrambled

- 1/4 cup chopped spinach
- 2 tablespoons crumbled feta cheese
- Salt and pepper to taste
- 1 teaspoon olive oil

Instructions:

- Heat olive oil in a skillet over medium heat.
- Add chopped spinach to the skillet and sauté for 1-2 minutes until wilted.
- Season scrambled eggs with salt and pepper, then add them to the skillet with the spinach.
- Cook, stirring occasionally, until eggs are set.
- Remove from heat and sprinkle crumbled feta cheese over the eggs.
- Warm the whole wheat tortilla in the skillet or microwave for a few seconds.
- Spoon the egg mixture onto the tortilla, then fold the sides in and roll it up.
- Serve warm.

Health Benefits:

➢ This breakfast wrap provides protein from eggs and healthy fats from feta cheese, along with vitamins and minerals from spinach.

➢ Whole wheat tortillas offer fiber and complex carbohydrates for sustained energy.

Preparation Time: 10 minutes

6. Berry Smoothie Bowl

Ingredients:

➢ 1/2 cup mixed berries (such as strawberries, blueberries, raspberries)

➢ 1/2 banana

➢ 1/2 cup spinach

➢ 1/2 cup unsweetened almond milk

➢ 1 tablespoon chia seeds

➢ Toppings: sliced banana, granola, shredded coconut, sliced almonds

Instructions:

➢ In a blender, combine mixed berries, banana, spinach, almond milk, and chia seeds.

27

- ➢ Blend until smooth and creamy.
- ➢ Pour the smoothie into a bowl.
- ➢ Top with sliced banana, granola, shredded coconut, and sliced almonds.
- ➢ Serve immediately.

Health Benefits:

- ➢ This smoothie bowl is packed with antioxidants, vitamins, and minerals from mixed berries, banana, and spinach.
- ➢ Chia seeds add fiber and healthy omega-3 fatty acids, while almond milk offers protein and healthy fats.

Preparation Time: 5 minutes

7. Sweet Potato Hash

Ingredients:

- ➢ 1 small sweet potato, peeled and diced
- ➢ 1/4 cup diced bell peppers
- ➢ 1/4 cup diced onions
- ➢ 1/4 teaspoon paprika
- ➢ 1/4 teaspoon garlic powder
- ➢ Salt and pepper to taste

- ➢ 1 tablespoon olive oil
- ➢ 1 egg (optional)

Instructions:

- ➢ Heat olive oil in a skillet over medium heat.
- ➢ Add diced sweet potato to the skillet and cook for 5-7 minutes until softened.
- ➢ Add diced bell peppers and onions to the skillet, along with paprika, garlic powder, salt, and pepper.
- ➢ Cook for another 5-7 minutes until vegetables are tender and lightly browned.
- ➢ Meanwhile, fry or poach an egg in a separate skillet if desired.
- ➢ Serve sweet potato hash topped with a cooked egg, if using.

Health Benefits:

- ➢ Sweet potatoes are rich in vitamins, minerals, and antioxidants, including beta-carotene, which supports thyroid health.
- ➢ Bell peppers and onions add flavor and additional nutrients to this hearty breakfast dish.

Preparation Time: 15 minutes

8. Avocado Toast with Smoked Salmon

Ingredients:

- ➤ 1 slice whole grain bread, toasted
- ➤ 1/2 ripe avocado, mashed
- ➤ 2 ounces smoked salmon
- ➤ 1 tablespoon chopped chives or green onions
- ➤ Lemon wedges (optional)
- ➤ Salt and pepper to taste

Instructions:

- ➤ Spread mashed avocado evenly onto the toasted whole grain bread.
- ➤ Top with smoked salmon and sprinkle chopped chives or green onions on top.
- ➤ Squeeze lemon juice over the avocado toast if desired.
- ➤ Season with salt and pepper to taste.
- ➤ Serve immediately.

Health Benefits:

➢ This avocado toast is packed with heart-healthy fats from avocado and omega-3 fatty acids from smoked salmon, which support brain health and inflammation reduction.

➢ Whole grain bread provides fiber and complex carbohydrates for sustained energy.

Preparation Time: 5 minutes

9. Cottage Cheese and Fruit Bowl

Ingredients:

➢ 1/2 cup low-fat cottage cheese
➢ 1/2 cup mixed fruit (such as berries, diced mango, kiwi)
➢ 1 tablespoon chopped nuts (such as almonds, walnuts)
➢ 1 teaspoon honey or maple syrup (optional)
➢ Pinch of cinnamon (optional)

Instructions:

➢ In a bowl, layer low-fat cottage cheese, mixed fruit, and chopped nuts.

- ➢ Drizzle honey or maple syrup on top if desired.
- ➢ Sprinkle cinnamon on top if desired.
- ➢ Serve immediately.

Health Benefits:

- ➢ Cottage cheese is a good source of protein and calcium, supporting muscle health and bone density.
- ➢ Mixed fruit adds natural sweetness and vitamins, while nuts offer healthy fats and crunch.

Preparation Time: 5 minutes

10. Chia Seed Pudding

Ingredients:

- ➢ 2 tablespoons chia seeds
- ➢ 1/2 cup unsweetened almond milk
- ➢ 1/2 teaspoon vanilla extract
- ➢ 1 teaspoon honey or maple syrup (optional)
- ➢ Toppings: sliced banana, berries, chopped nuts

Instructions:

- ➢ In a bowl or jar, combine chia seeds, almond milk, vanilla extract, and honey or maple syrup (if using).
- ➢ Stir well to combine.

- Cover and refrigerate for at least 2 hours or overnight, until the mixture thickens and forms a pudding-like consistency.
- Once the chia pudding is set, stir it well and transfer to a serving bowl.
- Top with sliced banana, berries, and chopped nuts.
- Serve chilled.

Health Benefits:

- Chia seeds are rich in fiber, omega-3 fatty acids, and antioxidants, supporting digestion, heart health, and inflammation reduction.
- Almond milk provides calcium and vitamin D, while honey or maple syrup adds natural sweetness.

Preparation Time: 5 minutes (plus chilling time)

11. Spinach and Mushroom Frittata

Ingredients:

- 4 eggs
- 1 cup chopped spinach
- 1/2 cup sliced mushrooms
- 1/4 cup diced onions

33

- 1/4 cup shredded mozzarella cheese
- Salt and pepper to taste
- 1 tablespoon olive oil

Instructions:

- Preheat the oven to 350°F (175°C).
- In a mixing bowl, beat the eggs and season with salt and pepper.
- Heat olive oil in an oven-safe skillet over medium heat.
- Sauté mushrooms and onions until softened, then add spinach and cook until wilted.
- Pour the beaten eggs over the vegetables in the skillet.
- Sprinkle shredded mozzarella cheese over the top.
- Transfer the skillet to the oven and bake for 12-15 minutes until the frittata is set and lightly golden.
- Slice into wedges and serve warm.

Health Benefits:

- This frittata is rich in protein from eggs and packed with vitamins and minerals from spinach, mushrooms, and onions, supporting thyroid health and overall nutrition.

Preparation Time: 20 minutes

12. Blueberry Almond Overnight Oats

Ingredients:

- ➤ 1/2 cup rolled oats
- ➤ 1/2 cup unsweetened almond milk
- ➤ 1/4 cup plain Greek yogurt
- ➤ 1/4 cup blueberries
- ➤ 1 tablespoon almond butter
- ➤ 1 teaspoon honey or maple syrup (optional)

Instructions:

- ➤ In a jar or container, combine rolled oats, almond milk, Greek yogurt, blueberries, almond butter, and honey or maple syrup (if using).
- ➤ Stir well to combine.
- ➤ Cover and refrigerate overnight.
- ➤ In the morning, give the oats a stir and enjoy cold or warm.

Health Benefits:

> This overnight oats recipe provides a balance of carbohydrates, protein, and healthy fats, along with antioxidants and fiber from blueberries and almond butter, supporting thyroid health and sustained energy levels.

Preparation Time: 5 minutes (plus overnight soaking)

13. Turkey Sausage Breakfast Skillet

Ingredients:

> 2 turkey sausage links, sliced
> 1/2 cup diced sweet potatoes
> 1/4 cup diced bell peppers
> 1/4 cup diced onions
> 1/4 teaspoon smoked paprika
> Salt and pepper to taste
> 1 tablespoon olive oil
> 2 eggs (optional)

Instructions:

> Heat olive oil in a skillet over medium heat.

➤ Add sliced turkey sausage links to the skillet and cook until browned.

➤ Add diced sweet potatoes, bell peppers, onions, smoked paprika, salt, and pepper to the skillet.

➤ Cook, stirring occasionally, until sweet potatoes are tender and lightly browned.

➤ Meanwhile, fry or poach eggs in a separate skillet if desired.

➤ Serve the turkey sausage breakfast skillet with cooked eggs on top, if using.

Health Benefits:

➤ This breakfast skillet is packed with protein from turkey sausage and provides complex carbohydrates and vitamins from sweet potatoes and vegetables, supporting thyroid health and providing sustained energy.

Preparation Time: 20 minutes

14. Apple Cinnamon Quinoa Porridge

Ingredients:

➤ 1/2 cup cooked quinoa

- 1/2 cup unsweetened almond milk
- 1/2 apple, diced
- 1 tablespoon chopped walnuts
- 1 teaspoon honey or maple syrup
- 1/4 teaspoon ground cinnamon

Instructions:

- In a saucepan, combine cooked quinoa and almond milk.
- Stir in diced apple, chopped walnuts, honey or maple syrup, and ground cinnamon.
- Cook over medium heat until heated through and slightly thickened, stirring occasionally.
- Serve warm.

Health Benefits:

- This quinoa porridge is rich in protein, fiber, and antioxidants, supporting thyroid health and providing sustained energy.
- Apples add natural sweetness and vitamins, while cinnamon offers flavor and additional health benefits.

Preparation Time: 10 minutes

15. Egg and Veggie Breakfast Muffins

Ingredients:

- 6 eggs
- 1/2 cup chopped spinach
- 1/4 cup diced bell peppers
- 1/4 cup diced tomatoes
- 1/4 cup shredded cheddar cheese
- Salt and pepper to taste
- Cooking spray

Instructions:

- Preheat the oven to 350°F (175°C). Grease a muffin tin with cooking spray.
- In a mixing bowl, beat the eggs and season with salt and pepper.
- Stir in chopped spinach, diced bell peppers, diced tomatoes, and shredded cheddar cheese.
- Pour the egg mixture evenly into the prepared muffin tin.
- Bake for 20-25 minutes until the egg muffins are set and lightly golden.

- Allow to cool slightly before removing from the muffin tin.
- Serve warm or refrigerate for later use.

Health Benefits:

- These egg and veggie breakfast muffins are a convenient and portable option rich in protein, vitamins, and minerals, supporting thyroid health and providing a satisfying breakfast option.

Preparation Time: 30 minutes

16. Peanut Butter Banana Smoothie

Ingredients:

- 1 ripe banana
- 2 tablespoons peanut butter
- 1/2 cup plain Greek yogurt
- 1/2 cup unsweetened almond milk
- 1 tablespoon honey or maple syrup (optional)
- Ice cubes (optional)

Instructions:

- In a blender, combine ripe banana, peanut butter, Greek yogurt, almond milk, honey or maple syrup (if using), and ice cubes (if using).
- Blend until smooth and creamy.
- Pour into glasses and serve immediately.

Health Benefits:

- This peanut butter banana smoothie provides protein, healthy fats, and complex carbohydrates, along with essential vitamins and minerals from banana and Greek yogurt, supporting thyroid health and providing sustained energy.

Preparation Time: 5 minutes

17. Egg and Avocado Breakfast Sandwich

Ingredients:

- 1 whole grain English muffin, toasted
- 1 egg, fried or scrambled
- 1/4 avocado, mashed
- 1 slice tomato
- Salt and pepper to taste

Instructions:

> ➤ Toast the whole grain English muffin until lightly golden.
> ➤ Cook the egg to your preference (fried or scrambled) and season with salt and pepper.
> ➤ Spread mashed avocado onto one half of the toasted English muffin.
> ➤ Top with cooked egg and a slice of tomato.
> ➤ Place the other half of the toasted English muffin on top to form a sandwich.
> ➤ Serve immediately.

Health Benefits:

> ➤ This breakfast sandwich is packed with protein, healthy fats, and fiber, supporting thyroid health and providing a satisfying and nutritious meal option.

Preparation Time: 10 minutes

18. Berry Protein Pancakes

Ingredients:

> ➤ 1/2 cup rolled oats
> ➤ 1/2 cup cottage cheese

- 2 eggs
- 1/2 teaspoon vanilla extract
- 1/2 cup mixed berries (such as strawberries, blueberries, raspberries)
- Cooking spray or butter

Instructions:

- In a blender, combine rolled oats, cottage cheese, eggs, and vanilla extract. Blend until smooth.
- Heat a non-stick skillet or griddle over medium heat and lightly coat with cooking spray or butter.
- Pour pancake batter onto the skillet to form small pancakes.
- Drop a few mixed berries onto each pancake.
- Cook until bubbles form on the surface, then flip and cook until golden brown on the other side.
- Repeat with the remaining batter.
- Serve warm with additional berries and a drizzle of honey or maple syrup if desired.

Health Benefits:

> ➢ These protein pancakes are rich in protein, fiber, and antioxidants, supporting thyroid health and providing a satisfying and nutrient-dense breakfast option.

Preparation Time: 15 minutes

19. Mediterranean Breakfast Bowl

Ingredients:

> ➢ 1/2 cup cooked quinoa
> ➢ 1/4 cup chickpeas, rinsed and drained
> ➢ 1/4 cup diced cucumber
> ➢ 1/4 cup diced tomatoes
> ➢ 1/4 cup chopped olives
> ➢ 1/4 cup crumbled feta cheese
> ➢ 1 tablespoon chopped fresh parsley
> ➢ 1 tablespoon extra virgin olive oil
> ➢ 1 tablespoon lemon juice
> ➢ Salt and pepper to taste

Instructions:

> In a bowl, combine cooked quinoa, chickpeas, diced cucumber, diced tomatoes, chopped olives, crumbled feta cheese, and chopped fresh parsley.
> Drizzle extra virgin olive oil and lemon juice over the top.
> Season with salt and pepper to taste.
> Toss well to combine.
> Serve at room temperature or chilled.

Health Benefits:

> This Mediterranean breakfast bowl is rich in protein, fiber, healthy fats, and antioxidants, supporting thyroid health and providing a refreshing and flavorful breakfast option.

Preparation Time: 15 minutes

20. Green Smoothie with Kale and Pineapple
Ingredients:

> 1 cup chopped kale leaves
> 1/2 cup chopped pineapple
> 1/2 banana

- 1/2 cup unsweetened almond milk
- 1/2 cup plain Greek yogurt
- 1 tablespoon chia seeds
- Honey or maple syrup to taste (optional)
- Ice cubes (optional)

Instructions:

- In a blender, combine chopped kale leaves, chopped pineapple, banana, almond milk, Greek yogurt, chia seeds, honey or maple syrup (if using), and ice cubes (if using).
- Blend until smooth and creamy.
- Pour into glasses and serve immediately.

Health Benefits:

- This green smoothie is packed with vitamins, minerals, fiber, and antioxidants from kale, pineapple, banana, and chia seeds, supporting thyroid health and providing a refreshing and nutritious breakfast option.

Preparation Time: 5 minutes

21. Berry Spinach Protein Smoothie

Ingredients:

- 1/2 cup mixed berries (such as strawberries, blueberries, raspberries)
- 1/2 cup spinach leaves
- 1/2 banana
- 1/2 cup plain Greek yogurt
- 1/2 cup unsweetened almond milk
- 1 tablespoon almond butter
- 1 teaspoon honey or maple syrup (optional)
- Ice cubes (optional)

Instructions:

- In a blender, combine mixed berries, spinach leaves, banana, Greek yogurt, almond milk, almond butter, honey or maple syrup (if using), and ice cubes (if using).
- Blend until smooth and creamy.
- Pour into glasses and serve immediately.

Health Benefits:

> This protein smoothie is packed with antioxidants, vitamins, and minerals from berries and spinach, while Greek yogurt and almond butter provide protein and healthy fats to support thyroid health and energy levels.

Preparation Time: 5 minutes

22. Turmeric Ginger Carrot Smoothie

Ingredients:

> 1/2 cup chopped carrots
> 1/2 inch fresh ginger, peeled
> 1/2 teaspoon ground turmeric
> 1/2 banana
> 1/2 cup plain Greek yogurt
> 1/2 cup unsweetened almond milk
> 1 tablespoon honey or maple syrup (optional)
> Ice cubes (optional)

Instructions:

> In a blender, combine chopped carrots, fresh ginger, ground turmeric, banana, Greek yogurt, almond milk, honey or maple syrup (if using), and ice cubes (if using).
> Blend until smooth and creamy.
> Pour into glasses and serve immediately.

Health Benefits:

> This turmeric ginger carrot smoothie is rich in antioxidants, anti-inflammatory compounds, and vitamins, supporting thyroid health and providing immune-boosting properties.

Preparation Time: 5 minutes

23. Salmon and Avocado Breakfast Bowl

Ingredients:

> 1/2 cup cooked quinoa
> 2 ounces smoked salmon
> 1/4 avocado, sliced
> 1/4 cup diced cucumber
> 1 tablespoon capers

- Lemon wedges
- Salt and pepper to taste

Instructions:

- In a bowl, layer cooked quinoa, smoked salmon, sliced avocado, diced cucumber, and capers.
- Squeeze lemon juice over the top.
- Season with salt and pepper to taste.
- Serve immediately.

Health Benefits:

- This breakfast bowl is rich in omega-3 fatty acids, protein, and healthy fats from smoked salmon and avocado, while quinoa provides fiber and essential nutrients to support thyroid health and overall well-being.

Preparation Time: 10 minutes

24. Chocolate Peanut Butter Protein Overnight Oats

Ingredients:

- 1/2 cup rolled oats

- 1/2 cup unsweetened almond milk
- 1 tablespoon cocoa powder
- 1 tablespoon peanut butter
- 1/2 banana, mashed
- 1 tablespoon honey or maple syrup
- 1 tablespoon chia seeds

Instructions:

- In a jar or container, combine rolled oats, almond milk, cocoa powder, peanut butter, mashed banana, honey or maple syrup, and chia seeds.
- Stir well to combine.
- Cover and refrigerate overnight.
- In the morning, give the oats a stir and enjoy cold or warm.

Health Benefits:

- These overnight oats are rich in protein, fiber, and antioxidants, with the added benefit of chocolate and peanut butter flavors to satisfy cravings while supporting thyroid health and providing sustained energy.

Preparation Time: 5 minutes (plus overnight soaking)

25. Veggie Breakfast Burrito

Ingredients:

- 1 whole grain tortilla
- 2 eggs, scrambled
- 1/4 cup black beans, drained and rinsed
- 1/4 cup diced bell peppers
- 1/4 cup diced onions
- 1/4 cup shredded cheese
- Salsa or avocado for topping (optional)
- Salt and pepper to taste

Instructions:

- Heat the whole grain tortilla in a skillet or microwave until warm.
- Fill the tortilla with scrambled eggs, black beans, diced bell peppers, diced onions, and shredded cheese.
- Roll up the tortilla to form a burrito.
- Serve with salsa or sliced avocado if desired.
- Season with salt and pepper to taste.
- Serve immediately.

Health Benefits:

> This veggie breakfast burrito is a balanced meal option rich in protein, fiber, vitamins, and minerals, supporting thyroid health and providing a satisfying and convenient breakfast option.

Preparation Time: 10 minutes

26. Mango Coconut Chia Pudding

Ingredients:

> 2 tablespoons chia seeds
> 1/2 cup unsweetened coconut milk
> 1/2 cup diced mango
> 1 tablespoon shredded coconut
> 1 teaspoon honey or maple syrup (optional)

Instructions:

> In a bowl or jar, combine chia seeds and coconut milk.
> Stir well to combine.
> Cover and refrigerate for at least 2 hours or overnight, until the mixture thickens and forms a pudding-like consistency.

➤ Once the chia pudding is set, stir in diced mango and shredded coconut.

➤ Drizzle honey or maple syrup over the top if desired.

➤ Serve chilled.

Health Benefits:

➤ This mango coconut chia pudding is rich in fiber, healthy fats, and antioxidants, supporting thyroid health and providing a delicious and refreshing breakfast option.

Preparation Time: 5 minutes (plus chilling time)

27. Banana Walnut Breakfast Cookies

Ingredients:

➤ 1 ripe banana, mashed

➤ 1/2 cup rolled oats

➤ 1/4 cup chopped walnuts

➤ 2 tablespoons almond butter

➤ 1 tablespoon honey or maple syrup

➤ 1/2 teaspoon ground cinnamon

➤ Pinch of salt

Instructions:

➢ Preheat the oven to 350°F (175°C). Line a baking sheet with parchment paper.

➢ In a mixing bowl, combine mashed banana, rolled oats, chopped walnuts, almond butter, honey or maple syrup, ground cinnamon, and a pinch of salt.

➢ Stir until well combined.

➢ Drop spoonfuls of the cookie dough onto the prepared baking sheet, shaping them into cookies.

➢ Bake for 12-15 minutes until lightly golden.

➢ Allow the cookies to cool on the baking sheet for a few minutes before transferring to a wire rack to cool completely.

➢ Serve at room temperature.

Health Benefits:

➢ These banana walnut breakfast cookies are a nutritious and convenient option rich in fiber, protein, and healthy fats, supporting thyroid health and providing a satisfying and portable breakfast option.

Preparation Time: 20 minutes

28. Mediterranean Egg Muffins

Ingredients:

- 6 eggs
- 1/4 cup diced tomatoes
- 1/4 cup chopped spinach
- 1/4 cup diced bell peppers
- 1/4 cup crumbled feta cheese
- Salt and pepper to taste
- Cooking spray

Instructions:

- Preheat the oven to 350°F (175°C). Grease a muffin tin with cooking spray.
- In a mixing bowl, beat the eggs and season with salt and pepper.
- Stir in diced tomatoes, chopped spinach, diced bell peppers, and crumbled feta cheese.
- Pour the egg mixture evenly into the prepared muffin tin.
- Bake for 20-25 minutes until the egg muffins are set and lightly golden.

- ➢ Allow to cool slightly before removing from the muffin tin.
- ➢ Serve warm or refrigerate for later use.

Health Benefits:

- ➢ These Mediterranean egg muffins are rich in protein, vitamins, and minerals, supporting thyroid health and providing a convenient and portable breakfast option.

Preparation Time: 30 minutes

29. Almond Flour Banana Pancakes

Ingredients:

- ➢ 1 ripe banana, mashed
- ➢ 2 eggs
- ➢ 1/2 teaspoon vanilla extract
- ➢ 1/2 cup almond flour
- ➢ 1/2 teaspoon baking powder
- ➢ Pinch of salt
- ➢ Cooking spray or butter

Instructions:

> ➤ In a mixing bowl, combine mashed banana, eggs, and vanilla extract. Mix until well combined.

> ➤ Stir in almond flour, baking powder, and a pinch of salt until a smooth batter forms.

> ➤ Heat a non-stick skillet or griddle over medium heat and lightly coat with cooking spray or butter.

> ➤ Pour pancake batter onto the skillet to form small pancakes.

> ➤ Cook until bubbles form on the surface, then flip and cook until golden brown on the other side.

> ➤ Repeat with the remaining batter.

> ➤ Serve warm with toppings of your choice, such as sliced bananas, berries, or a drizzle of honey or maple syrup.

Health Benefits:

> ➤ These almond flour banana pancakes are gluten-free, grain-free, and rich in protein, fiber, and healthy fats, supporting thyroid health and providing a delicious and nutritious breakfast option.

Preparation Time: 15 minutes

30. Tomato Basil Avocado Toast

Ingredients:

- ➤ 1 slice whole grain bread, toasted
- ➤ 1/4 avocado, mashed
- ➤ 1/2 cup cherry tomatoes, sliced
- ➤ Fresh basil leaves
- ➤ Balsamic glaze (optional)
- ➤ Salt and pepper to taste

Instructions:

- ➤ Spread mashed avocado evenly onto the toasted whole grain bread.
- ➤ Top with sliced cherry tomatoes and fresh basil leaves.
- ➤ Drizzle with balsamic glaze if desired.
- ➤ Season with salt and pepper to taste.
- ➤ Serve immediately.

Health Benefits:

- ➤ This tomato basil avocado toast is a flavorful and nutrient-rich breakfast option rich in healthy fats, vitamins, and antioxidants, supporting thyroid health and providing a satisfying meal to start the day.

Preparation Time: 5 minutes

31. Green Tea Matcha Smoothie

Ingredients:

- ➤ 1/2 cup brewed green tea, cooled
- ➤ 1/2 banana
- ➤ 1/2 cup spinach leaves
- ➤ 1/4 avocado
- ➤ 1 tablespoon plain Greek yogurt
- ➤ 1 teaspoon matcha powder
- ➤ 1 teaspoon honey or maple syrup (optional)
- ➤ Ice cubes (optional)

Instructions:

- ➤ In a blender, combine brewed green tea, banana, spinach leaves, avocado, Greek yogurt, matcha powder, honey or maple syrup (if using), and ice cubes (if using).
- ➤ Blend until smooth and creamy.
- ➤ Pour into glasses and serve immediately.

Health Benefits:

➢ This green tea matcha smoothie is rich in antioxidants, vitamins, and minerals from green tea, spinach, avocado, and matcha powder, supporting thyroid health and providing a refreshing and energizing breakfast option.

Preparation Time: 5 minutes

32. Chia Seed Breakfast Bowl

Ingredients:

➢ 2 tablespoons chia seeds
➢ 1/2 cup unsweetened almond milk
➢ 1/2 teaspoon vanilla extract
➢ 1/2 cup mixed berries (such as strawberries, blueberries, raspberries)
➢ 1 tablespoon sliced almonds
➢ 1 teaspoon honey or maple syrup (optional)

Instructions:

➢ In a bowl or jar, combine chia seeds, almond milk, and vanilla extract.
➢ Stir well to combine.

- Cover and refrigerate for at least 2 hours or overnight, until the mixture thickens and forms a pudding-like consistency.
- Once the chia pudding is set, stir in mixed berries and sliced almonds.
- Drizzle honey or maple syrup over the top if desired.
- Serve chilled.

Health Benefits:

- This chia seed breakfast bowl is rich in fiber, protein, healthy fats, and antioxidants, supporting thyroid health and providing a delicious and nutritious breakfast option.

Preparation Time: 5 minutes (plus chilling time)

33. Veggie Breakfast Wrap with Hummus

Ingredients:

- 1 whole grain tortilla
- 2 tablespoons hummus
- 1/4 cup chopped spinach
- 1/4 cup diced tomatoes
- 1/4 cup sliced cucumber

- ➤ 2 tablespoons crumbled feta cheese
- ➤ Salt and pepper to taste

Instructions:

- ➤ Spread hummus evenly onto the whole grain tortilla.
- ➤ Top with chopped spinach, diced tomatoes, sliced cucumber, and crumbled feta cheese.
- ➤ Season with salt and pepper to taste.
- ➤ Roll up the tortilla to form a wrap.
- ➤ Serve immediately.

Health Benefits:

- ➤ This veggie breakfast wrap is packed with fiber, vitamins, minerals, and antioxidants from vegetables, along with protein and healthy fats from hummus and feta cheese, supporting thyroid health and providing a satisfying and nutritious breakfast option.

Preparation Time: 10 minutes

34. Peanut Butter Banana Protein Shake

Ingredients:

- ➤ 1 ripe banana

- 1 tablespoon peanut butter
- 1/2 cup plain Greek yogurt
- 1/2 cup unsweetened almond milk
- 1 scoop protein powder (vanilla or chocolate flavor)
- Ice cubes (optional)

Instructions:

- In a blender, combine ripe banana, peanut butter, Greek yogurt, almond milk, protein powder, and ice cubes (if using).
- Blend until smooth and creamy.
- Pour into glasses and serve immediately.

Health Benefits:

- This peanut butter banana protein shake is rich in protein, healthy fats, and carbohydrates, supporting thyroid health and providing a satisfying and energizing breakfast option.

Preparation Time: 5 minutes

35. Cauliflower Hash Browns

Ingredients:

- 1 cup grated cauliflower

- ➤ 1 egg
- ➤ 2 tablespoons almond flour
- ➤ 1/4 teaspoon garlic powder
- ➤ 1/4 teaspoon onion powder
- ➤ Salt and pepper to taste
- ➤ Cooking spray or olive oil

Instructions:

- ➤ In a mixing bowl, combine grated cauliflower, egg, almond flour, garlic powder, onion powder, salt, and pepper. Mix until well combined.
- ➤ Heat cooking spray or olive oil in a skillet over medium heat.
- ➤ Drop spoonfuls of the cauliflower mixture onto the skillet and flatten with a spatula to form hash browns.
- ➤ Cook for 3-4 minutes on each side until golden brown and crispy.
- ➤ Serve hot.

Health Benefits:

- ➤ These cauliflower hash browns are a low-carb alternative to traditional hash browns, providing fiber, vitamins, and minerals from cauliflower, along with protein and healthy fats from egg and almond flour, supporting thyroid health and providing a delicious and nutritious breakfast option.

Preparation Time: 15 minutes

36. Strawberry Almond Breakfast Quinoa

Ingredients:

- 1/2 cup cooked quinoa
- 1/2 cup sliced strawberries
- 2 tablespoons sliced almonds
- 1 tablespoon honey or maple syrup
- 1/2 teaspoon vanilla extract
- Pinch of cinnamon

Instructions:

- In a bowl, combine cooked quinoa, sliced strawberries, sliced almonds, honey or maple syrup, vanilla extract, and a pinch of cinnamon.
- Stir well to combine.
- Serve warm or chilled.

Health Benefits:

> This strawberry almond breakfast quinoa is rich in protein, fiber, vitamins, and minerals, supporting thyroid health and providing a satisfying and nutrient-dense breakfast option.

Preparation Time: 10 minutes

37. Mediterranean Egg White Frittata

Ingredients:

> 4 egg whites
> 1/4 cup diced tomatoes
> 1/4 cup chopped spinach
> 1/4 cup sliced black olives
> 1/4 cup crumbled feta cheese
> Salt and pepper to taste
> Cooking spray or olive oil

Instructions:

> Preheat the oven to 350°F (175°C). Grease a small oven-safe skillet with cooking spray or olive oil.

- In a mixing bowl, whisk together egg whites, diced tomatoes, chopped spinach, sliced black olives, crumbled feta cheese, salt, and pepper.
- Pour the egg mixture into the greased skillet.
- Bake for 15-20 minutes until the frittata is set and lightly golden.
- Allow to cool slightly before slicing.
- Serve warm.

Health Benefits:

- This Mediterranean egg white frittata is low in calories and fat, rich in protein, vitamins, and minerals, supporting thyroid health and providing a delicious and nutritious breakfast option.

Preparation Time: 20 minutes

38. Coconut Yogurt Parfait

Ingredients:

- 1/2 cup coconut yogurt
- 1/4 cup granola
- 1/4 cup mixed berries (such as strawberries, blueberries, raspberries)

- ➤ 1 tablespoon shredded coconut
- ➤ Drizzle of honey or maple syrup (optional)

Instructions:

- ➤ In a glass or jar, layer coconut yogurt, granola, mixed berries, and shredded coconut.
- ➤ Drizzle with honey or maple syrup if desired.
- ➤ Serve immediately.

Health Benefits:

- ➤ This coconut yogurt parfait is rich in probiotics, fiber, antioxidants, and healthy fats, supporting thyroid health and providing a delicious and refreshing breakfast option.

Preparation Time: 5 minutes

39. Quinoa Breakfast Bowl with Poached Egg

Ingredients:

- ➤ 1/2 cup cooked quinoa
- ➤ 1 poached egg
- ➤ 1/4 avocado, sliced
- ➤ 1/4 cup cherry tomatoes, halved
- ➤ 1 tablespoon chopped fresh cilantro

> 1 teaspoon olive oil

> Salt and pepper to taste

Instructions:

> In a bowl, combine cooked quinoa, poached egg, sliced avocado, cherry tomatoes, chopped fresh cilantro, olive oil, salt, and pepper.

> Toss well to combine.

> Serve warm.

Health Benefits:

> This quinoa breakfast bowl is rich in protein, fiber, vitamins, and minerals, supporting thyroid health and providing a satisfying and nutrient-dense breakfast option.

Preparation Time: 15 minutes

40. Pumpkin Spice Chia Pudding

Ingredients:

> 2 tablespoons chia seeds

> 1/2 cup unsweetened almond milk

> 1/4 cup pumpkin puree

> 1 tablespoon maple syrup

- 1/4 teaspoon pumpkin pie spice
- 1 tablespoon chopped pecans (optional)

Instructions:

- In a bowl or jar, combine chia seeds, almond milk, pumpkin puree, maple syrup, and pumpkin pie spice.
- Stir well to combine.
- Cover and refrigerate for at least 2 hours or overnight, until the mixture thickens and forms a pudding-like consistency.
- Once the chia pudding is set, stir well and transfer to a serving bowl.
- Top with chopped pecans if desired.
- Serve chilled.

Health Benefits:

- This pumpkin spice chia pudding is rich in fiber, vitamins, and minerals, with the added benefit of pumpkin puree and warming spices, supporting thyroid health and providing a delicious and seasonal breakfast option.

Preparation Time: 5 minutes (plus chilling time)

CONCLUSION

Embarking on a journey to manage hypothyroidism through dietary adjustments is not merely about following a set of recipes; it's about embracing a lifestyle that prioritizes nourishment, balance, and well-being.

This cookbook for beginners serves as a guiding light, offering not just recipes, but a roadmap to better health.

As you explore the pages of this cookbook, may you discover the power of wholesome ingredients, the joy of preparing nourishing meals, and the profound impact that mindful eating can have on your overall health.

Remember, each recipe is crafted with care and consideration, tailored to support your thyroid health while tantalizing your taste buds.

But beyond the kitchen, let this cookbook be a reminder that taking control of your health is within your reach.

With each meal, you're not just feeding your body; you're fueling your journey toward vitality and well-being.

So, whether you're just starting out on your hypothyroidism diet or you're a seasoned pro seeking new culinary adventures, may this cookbook be your trusted companion.

Here's to savoring the flavors of good health, one delicious bite at a time.

Embrace the journey, nourish your body, and thrive.

Your health is in your hands, and with this cookbook, you have all the tools you need to make every meal a step toward a happier, healthier you.

Made in the USA
Middletown, DE
20 July 2025